Vedimar Cabral Oliveira

Phototherapy in Newborns

Vedimar Cabral Oliveira

Phototherapy in Newborns

Care for newborns undergoing phototherapy treatment

ScienciaScripts

Imprint

Any brand names and product names mentioned in this book are subject to trademark, brand or patent protection and are trademarks or registered trademarks of their respective holders. The use of brand names, product names, common names, trade names, product descriptions etc. even without a particular marking in this work is in no way to be construed to mean that such names may be regarded as unrestricted in respect of trademark and brand protection legislation and could thus be used by anyone.

Cover image: www.ingimage.com

This book is a translation from the original published under ISBN 978-613-9-72068-2.

Publisher:
Sciencia Scripts
is a trademark of
Dodo Books Indian Ocean Ltd. and OmniScriptum S.R.L publishing group

120 High Road, East Finchley, London, N2 9ED, United Kingdom
Str. Armeneasca 28/1, office 1, Chisinau MD-2012, Republic of Moldova, Europe
Printed at: see last page
ISBN: 978-620-7-72647-9

Thank you

In particular, I thank God for giving me the health and strength to overcome difficulties.

And to everyone who, directly or indirectly, contributed to the realisation, not only of this work, but of this new stage in my life.

Dedication

To my eternal boyfriend: José Fernandes for believing in my potential;

To my brother: Valdenor Cabral, for his support and strength.

To my daughter: Ana Lydia for understanding my absence.

And to my supervisor: Mª MARISLEI ESPÍNDULA for her patience and dedication.

Epigraph

"I chose shifts because I know that the dark of night frightens the sick. I chose to
be present in pain because I've been so close to suffering. I chose to serve my
neighbour because I know that we all need help one day.
I chose white because I want to convey peace. I chose to study working
methods because books are a source of knowledge.
I chose to be a nurse because I love and respect life! "

(FLORENCE NIGHTINGALE 1820-19

SUMMARY

SUMMARY

OLIVEIRA, Vedimar Cabral. *Nursing Care for Newborns Treated with Phototherapy.* Integrative Review. Goiânia: Centre for Nursing and Nutrition Studies/PUC-GO; 2017.

The aim of this study was to search the literature for scientific evidence on nursing care for newborns undergoing phototherapy. The method used consisted of an integrative review of 20 articles located in the SCIELO and LILACS electronic library databases. The results showed that the role of nursing is indispensable in the knowledge of these procedures in order not only to fulfil the prescription but also to care for the jaundiced newborn with knowledge, safety, efficiency and special care to achieve the results. The study leads to the conclusion that nursing has a wide-ranging role, from fully identifying the components, handling, choosing, adapting, adjusting and measuring the irradiance of phototherapy devices with or without the baby, to specifically caring for the newborn undergoing phototherapy treatment in order to obtain the best results in the shortest time and with the minimum acceptable side effects in this practice.

Keywords: Phototherapy; Newborns; Nursing; Jaundice.

1- INTRODUCTION

The interest or motivation to research *nursing care for newborns undergoing phototherapy* arose from the observation that there is a high incidence of newborns being born with jaundice. This occurs basically when there is an excessive production of bilirubin and/or when there is a deficient elimination of it.

Neonatal jaundice or jaundice of the newborn is a common condition, especially in babies born before 36 weeks, and is a normal and expected phenomenon. Indirect bilirubin levels in newborns are naturally higher than in adults. Phototherapy is the most common treatment used to lower bilirubin levels. Jaundice, which is characterised by the yellowing of the skin, sclera and nails, caused by an excessive level of bilirubin accumulated in the blood (NEWMAN *et al,* 2009).

Jaundice is classified as physiological or pathological, with physiological jaundice being characterised by its appearance after 24 hours of life. Pathological jaundice, on the other hand, appears within the first 24 hours of life, showing an underlying disorder of potential severity, characterised by a rapid increase in serum total bilirubin levels (HINKES, CLOHERTY, 2000; OLIVEIRA, 2006).

Phototherapy is currently the first choice for treating jaundice, as it is a non-invasive and very effective method. It includes conventional phototherapy, dichroic halogen (bilispot®), high-intensity reflective phototherapy (biliberço®), high-intensity phototherapy (bilitron®) and iodine emission (COLVERO; COLVERO; FIORI, 2005; CORREA; TOMASI, 2007; NEWMAN et al, 2009).

Phototherapy is the therapeutic modality that applies repeated and controlled exposures of ultraviolet radiation to alter skin physiology in order to induce regression or control the evolution of various dermatoses. It is used to treat various skin diseases such as psoriasis, vitiligo, cutaneous T-cell lymphoma, topical dermatitis, universal alopecia, nodular pruritus, renal pruritus, scleroderma and other dermatoses (TEIXEIRA et al., 1997).

Nursing has a wide-ranging role, from complete identification of the components, handling, choosing, adapting, adjusting and measuring the irradiance of the devices with or without the baby, to specific care for the newborn undergoing phototherapy treatment in order to obtain the best results, in the shortest time and with the fewest acceptable side effects in this practice (GAÍVA, GOMES, 2003).

The work carried out lies in the fact that the role of nursing is indispensable in the knowledge of these procedures in order not only to fulfil the prescription but also to care for the jaundiced newborn with knowledge, safety, efficiency and special care to achieve the results.

2- OBJECTIVE

To search the literature for scientific evidence on nursing care for newborns undergoing phototherapy.

3- METHODOLOGY

This is a descriptive study carried out using the integrative review method, the aim of which is to summarise knowledge on the use of phototherapy in newborns, as well as to produce new knowledge that has not been addressed or deepened in previous research. It should be noted that an integrative review carried out effectively requires the same standards of rigour, clarity and replication used in primary studies (COOPER, 1984).

The guiding question to answer the research objective was: what *nursing care is given to newborns undergoing phototherapy treatments?*

The bibliographic search took place in the Scientific Electronic Library Online (SciELO) and LILACS databases, where the following descriptors were used according to their definition in the DeCS (Health Sciences Descriptors) (Chart 1): phototherapy in newborns, neonatal jaundice and nursing care with phototherapy. The SciELO search strategy used the descriptors "phototherapy in newborns" and "neonatal jaundice", and 16 publications were found. The LILACS database used the descriptors "nursing care with phototherapy" and found 3 publications. Different forms and quantities of keywords were used in each database due to the definitions that each database proposes for the descriptors and different terms were used in the search field of each database, such as words and subject descriptors. With this procedure, it is possible that a greater number of articles related to the topic of interest were captured in each database.

Chart 1: Systematisation of the electronic search.

Database	Descriptors	Articles found	Selected articles	Final sample
SciELO	"Phototherapy in newborns" and "Neonatal jaundice"	20	16	12
LILACS	"Nursing care with phototherapy"	6	4	2
	TOTAL	26	20	14

The inclusion criteria were: research available in full in the selected databases in Portuguese, English or Spanish, whose results favoured the treatment of phototherapy in newborns.

Publications that dealt with nursing care for newborns in a generalised way were excluded, as they did not meet the proposed theme.

4- RESULTS

The sample consisted of 14 articles, all of which were retrospective studies in Portuguese. The papers were published between 1995 and 2010 in Brazilian journals (Chart 2).

Chart 2: Distribution of phototherapy studies according to study identification, year of publication, type of study, objectives and main results.

Identification of the study (Title, authors, journal)	Year of Publication	Base of Data	Type of Study	Objectives
Educational technology for the practice of nursing care with mothers of neonates under phototherapy. Campos ACS, Cardoso MVLML. TextoContexto Nursing.	2008	SciELO	Retrospective Study	Describe the use of atechnology education in the practice of care nursing with mothers of neonates using phototherapy
Nursing and humanistic care: an intervention proposal for the mother of a newborn under phototherapy. Campos ACS, Cardoso MVLML. Science and Nursing.	2006	SciELO	Retrospective Study	Describe nursing interventions based strategies and techniques for communicating with the mother of a neonate undergoing phototherapy
Indications of phototherapy in term newborns with non-hemolytic jaundice: a critical analysis. Carvalho M, Lopes JMA. Jornalde Paediatrics.	1995	LILACS	Retrospective Study	To critically analyse the use of phototherapy and propose practical parameters to help paediatricians decide whether to treat a full-term newborn with non-hemolytic hyperbilirubinaemia.

Caring for newborns undergoing phototherapy: the knowledge of the nursing team. Gomes NS, Teixeira JBA, Barichello E. Revista Eletronica de Enfermagem.	2010	LILACS	Retrospective Study	Identifying knowledge of nursing staff about caring for newbornsand complications related to phototherapy.
Communication: a basic nursing tool for caring for the mother of a newborn under phototherapy.Campos ACS, Cardoso MVLM, Pagliuca LMF, Rossi LA. Journal of the Nursing Network North-East.	2008	LILACS	Retrospective Study	To understand the communication process between the health team and the mothers of neonates under phototherapy in the light of the assumptions of Humanistic Theory.
Development of an eye protector for phototherapy in newborns: a technology. Silva L, Silva FS, Turiani M, Juliani CMCM, Spiri WC. Revista Latino Enfermagem.	2008	SciELO	Retrospective Study	Describe development of an invention (patented utility model) for the protection of newborns undergoing phototherapy
Evaluation of the clinical efficacy of a new modality phototherapy using light-emitting diodes.	2007	SciELO	Retrospective Study	Evaluate the therapeutic efficacy of a microprocessor-based phototherapy system that utilises the

Martins BMR, Carvalho M, Moreira MEL, Lopes JMA.Jornalde Paediatrics.				high-intensity light-emitting diodes (Super LEDs) treatment of hyperbilirubinaemia in premature newborns.
Polymers Luminescents as Non-Ionising Radiation Sensors: Application in Phototherapy Neonatal. Vasconcelos CKB, Bianchi RF. Institute of Exact and Biological Sciences.	2007	SciELO	Retrospective Study	Demonstrate the possibility of using luminescent systems as an active element in non-ionising radiation detectors, especially in the region used to detect non-ionising radiation. prophylaxis and phototherapy treatment of neonatal hyperbilirubinaemia.
When should we start phototherapy in preterm newborns? Almeida MFB. Journal of Paediatrics.	2004	SciELO	Retrospective Study	Demonstrate the appropriate time to start treatment phototherapy in newborns.
Educational technology for the practice of nursing care with mothers of neonates under phototherapy. Campos ACS, Cardoso MVLML. TextoContexto	2008	SciELO	Retrospective Study	Describe the use of a technology education in the practice of care nursing with mothers of neonates undergoing phototherapy.

Nursing.				
Maternal perceptions of neonates undergoing phototherapy. Rodrigues FLS, Silveira IP, Campos ACS. Anna Nery School.	2007	SciELO	Retrospective Study	Find out about mothers' perceptions of phototherapy and identify their difficulties related to it. phototherapy treatment.
Application of the Paterson and Zderad theory with mothers of newborns under phototherapy. Campos ACS, Cardoso MVLML. TextoContexto Nursing.	2004	SciELO	Retrospective Study	Applying the humanistic theory of Paterson and Zderad with mothers of newborn babies (NB) under phototherapy.
Phototherapy. Duarte I, Buense R, Kobata C. Brazilian Annals of Demartology.	2006	SciELO	Retrospective Study	Present some limitations, such as the need specific equipment, patient compliance , the possibility of indication to the patient and the cumulative dose of UV irradiation.

The use of phototherapy in newborns: evaluation of clinical practice. Vieira AA, Lima CLMA, Carvalho M, Moreira MEL. <u>Brazilian Journal of Maternal and Child Health</u>	2004	SciELO	Retrospective Study	Describe the use of phototherapy in daily clinical practice by health professionals in maternity hospitals in the city of Rio de Janeiro.

5- DISCUSSION

Some problems are common in the neonatal period, and one of the most common is jaundice.

In addition to prematurity and low birth weight, some clinical situations predispose newborns to jaundice, such as cases of blood incompatibility between mother and baby, maternal use of oxytocin and diazepam, and traumatic births with cephalohematoma or other bleeding, as this increases the degradation of haemoglobin and consequently the formation of bilirubin. (SILVA, 2002; BUENO, SACAI, TOMA, 2003; ALMEIDA, 2004; COLVERO, COLVERO, FIORI, 2005; OLIVEIRA, 2005; PETROVA et al, 2006; TAMEZ, SILVA, 2006).

Jaundice is classified as physiological or pathological, with physiological jaundice being characterised by its appearance after 24 hours of life. Pathological jaundice presents itself within the first 24 hours of life, showing an underlying disorder of potential severity, characterised by a rapid increase in serum total bilirubin levels (HINKES, CLOHERTY, 2000; OLIVEIRA, 2006).

It is possible to prevent or treat hyperbilirubinaemia by exposing the newborn to light with a wavelength of approximately 450nm. The light rays transform bilirubin IX alpha into a relatively stable geometric isomer through a photochemical process (GAIVA, 2003).

When used correctly, phototherapy controls bilirubin levels in almost all patients, with the exception of those with severe haemolytic conditions and low birth weight newborns (under 1,500g) with extensive haematomas.(ALMEIDA, 2004)

The phototherapy procedure consists of exposing the child to a light source for hours or days; in this case, newborns remain in their cots, wearing only a nappy and blindfold, subjected to the light coming from seven fluorescent lamps or 14 lamps, half placed above and half below the baby in the double phototherapy units.

The light converts the bilirubin impregnated in the skin and mucous membranes into another substance, preventing it from accumulating in the brain (GAIVA, 2003).

Newborn care is divided into immediate and general care. Immediate care is the care that the team must take in the delivery room to maintain the life of the newborn and avoid future sequelae, while general care is care during the neonatal period, when the child is adapting to life outside the womb (ARONE, 2003).

Nursing has a wide-ranging role, from fully identifying the components, handling, choosing, adapting, adjusting and measuring the irradiance of the devices with or without the baby, to specifically caring for the newborn undergoing phototherapy in order to obtain the best results, in the shortest time and with the fewest acceptable side effects in this practice.

Few clinical trials were found on the researched problem, especially on treatment without phototherapy, demonstrating the need to carry out studies with designs that can collaborate in providing strong evidence for a good prognosis for newborns with jaundice.

Neonatal jaundice

Some problems are common in the neonatal period, and one of the most common is jaundice (CORREA, TOMASI, 2007).

The incidence of jaundice in newborns varies between authors, ranging from 25 to 50 per cent in term newborns, and this percentage is even higher in preterm newborns (PTNB) (OLIVEIRA, 2005). Almeida (2004) adds that hyperbilirubinaemia is found in practically all PTNBs, especially very low birth weight ones. Some of these newborns need intensive care to treat jaundice, requiring hospitalisation in neonatal units.

In addition to prematurity and low birth weight, some clinical situations predispose newborns to jaundice, such as cases of blood incompatibility between mother and baby, maternal use of Oxytocin and Diazepam and traumatic birth with cephalohematoma or other bleeding, as this increases the degradation of haemoglobin and consequently the formation of bilirubin (SILVA, 2002; BUENO, SACAI, TOMA, 2003; ALMEIDA, 2004; COLVERO, COLVERO, FIORI, 2005; OLIVEIRA, 2005; PETROVA et al, 2006; TAMEZ, SILVA, 2006).

Jaundice is classified as physiological or pathological, with physiological jaundice being characterised by its appearance after 24 hours of life. Pathological jaundice appears in the first 24 hours of life, showing an underlying disorder of potential severity, characterised by a rapid increase in serum total bilirubin levels (HINKES, CLOHERTY, 2000; OLIVEIRA, 2006).

Physiological jaundice

According to Lowdermilk, Perry and Bobak (2002), physiological jaundice occurs in 50 per cent of term newborns (at 40 weeks) and 80 per cent of premature newborns. Neonatal jaundice occurs because the newborn has a higher level of bilirubin production. The number of foetal red blood cells per kilo of body weight in newborns is higher than in adults.

According to Silva (2008), physiological jaundice is characterised by an increase in indirect bilirubin levels, reaching a rate of 7 mg/dl around day 3^a of life.

Physiological jaundice, according to Lowdermilk, Perry and Bobak (2002),

> It is usually seen first on the head, sclera and mucous membranes, gradually progressing to the chest, abdomen and extremities. According to the authors, various hospital practices influence the appearance and degree of physiological hyperbilirubinaemia (LOWDERMILK, PERRY and BOBAK, 2002, p. 502).

Pathological jaundice

Pathological jaundice manifests itself in the first 24 hours of life and persists for up to a week (BUENO et al., 2003).

According to Lowdermilk, Perry and Bobak (2002), there are many possible causes of pathological hyperbilirubinaemia in neonates. The most common is incompatibility between maternal and foetal blood, specifically ABO and Rh incompatibility. ABO incompatibility is more common than Rh incompatibility, but causes less serious problems in the affected newborn.

According to Santos et al. (2002) it can be characterised as:

- Jaundice beginning in the first 24 hours of life;

- Increased direct and indirect bilirubin, with normal values: BD:0.3 mg/dl and BI: 1 mg/dl;

According to Segre (2002):

- In term NB, hyperbilirubinaemia with values above 12 mg/dl, and premature NB, values above 15 mg/dl;

- Persistent jaundice beyond the first week of life;

- Jaundice with increased direct bilirubin of 1 to 2 mg/dl

With the increase in circulating bilirubin, the newborn may progressively manifest (SANTOS et al., 2002):

- Weak suction

- Hypoactivity

- Hepatosplenomegaly

- Anaemia

- Anasarca

- Kernicterus

Phototherapy

According to Arone (2003), the first studies on the effects of light on bilirubin metabolism were carried out in 1958 by Dr RJ Cremer, considered the father of phototherapy.

The use of phototherapy treatment in Brazil began in 1960, mirroring the English model, through haematologist Dr Humberto Costa Ferreira, from the São Paulo Medical School (RODRIGUES et al., 2007).

According to Arone (2003), phototherapy is indicated for reducing serum levels of indirect bilirubin in jaundiced newborns, and requires care due to the risks of hyperbilirubinaemia at this stage of life, when indirect bilirubin toxicity requires intervention due to the irreversible neurological sequelae it can produce.

It is possible to prevent or treat hyperbilirubinaemia by exposing the newborn to light with a wavelength of around 450nm. It seems that light rays transform bilirubin IX alpha into a relatively stable geometric isomer through a photochemical process (SHERLOCK, 1985).

When used correctly, phototherapy controls bilirubin levels in almost all patients, with the exception of those with severe haemolytic conditions and very low birth weight NBs (under 1,500g) with extensive haematomas (SMP, 2005; PEREIRA 2009).

Phototherapy Efficiency - Radiance

Phototherapy is currently the first choice for treating jaundice, as it is a non-invasive and very effective method. Types of phototherapy include conventional phototherapy, dichroic halogen phototherapy (bilispot®), high-intensity reflective phototherapy (biliberço®), high-intensity phototherapy (bilitron®) and iodine emission phototherapy (COLVERO; COLVERO; FIORI, 2005; CORREA;

TOMASI, 2007; NEWMAN et al, 2009).

The effectiveness of phototherapy treatment will depend on factors such as the irradiance of the light source, the spectrum of the light emitted, the length of time the lamps are used, the distance of the neonate from the light source, the area of the body surface exposed to the light, as well as the initial bilirubin concentration (FACCHINI, 2001; BUENO; SACAI; TOMA, 2003; OLIVEIRA, 2005; COLVERO; COLVERO; FIORI, 2005).

According to Barbosa (1988):

> Although any area of the skin results in the production of photoisomerised bilirubin, areas of the skin that are covered during phototherapy are not lightened and remain visibly jaundiced, reducing the effectiveness of phototherapy. (BARBOSA, 1988, p. 127)

According to Almeida (2008), the main aim in treating jaundice is to prevent the accumulation of bilirubin in the brain, which can cause major problems for the child's development. When a treatable cause of jaundice is identified, this specific treatment is extremely important.

The phototherapy procedure consists of exposing the child to a light source for hours or days; in this case, newborns remain in their cots, wearing only a nappy and blindfold, subjected to the light coming from seven fluorescent lamps or 14 lamps, half placed above and half below the baby in the double phototherapy units. The light converts bilirubin, which is impregnated in the skin and mucous membranes, into another substance, preventing it from accumulating in the brain (Carvalho apud CORREA and TOMASI, 2008).

It has been described that the routine use of blue light can cause the therapy administrator to have difficulty observing the child's colour, dizziness, vomiting and be painful to the eyes, which is why they are not popular in phototherapy systems. The combination of blue and white lights has been used with the advantage of minimising the problems with blue light (ARONE, 2003).

According to Carvalho (2001), the success of phototherapy depends on the photochemical transformation of bilirubin in the areas exposed to light. These reactions alter the structure of the bilirubin molecule and allow the photoproducts to be eliminated by the kidneys or liver without undergoing metabolic changes. Therefore, the basic mechanism of action of phototherapy is the utilisation of light energy in the transformation of bilirubin and more water-soluble products. Bilirubin absorbs light around 400 to 500nm. The light emitted in this range penetrates the epidermis and reaches the subcutaneous tissue. As a result, only bilirubin that is close to the surface of the skin (up to 2mm) will be directly affected by the light.

According to Mello (2004), two mechanisms have been proposed to explain the action of phototherapy in reducing serum bilirubin a levels:

-Photoisomerisation: this is the most important; it causes the transformation of bilirubin into lumirubin, which is soluble in water and rapidly excreted by the liver and kidneys without the need for conjugation.

Photo-oxidation: the conversion of bilirubin into small, water-soluble polar products that can be excreted in the urine.

The **Use of Phototherapy**

Although the beneficial effects outweigh those of not using it, phototherapy is not without its risks and can cause dehydration due to the insensitive loss of water, an increase in the number of bowel movements, lethargy, erythema, tanning, burns and retinal damage (BUENO, SACAI, TOMA, 2003; ASKIN, WILSON, 2006; TAMEZ, SILVA, 2006). Therefore, certain precautions are essential during phototherapy so that it can take place effectively and without causing consequences for the newborn.

According to Almeida (2004):

> Phototherapy should be used whenever the serum level of indirect bilirubin is a factor capable of exposing the newborn to the danger of toxic levels, whatever the aetiology. It is clear that situations that are not dependent on direct hyperbilirubinaemia or those in which haemolysis is intense are the ones that have the greatest indication (ALMEIDA, 2004, p. 246).

In cases of Rh and sometimes ABO incompatibility, phototherapy will be used as an adjunct and exsanguineotransfusion the most appropriate treatment (BARBOSA, 1988).

The intermittent use of phototherapy has been shown to be more effective than its continuous use, since it has been observed that it is in the first few hours after starting each period of exposure that there is a greater decrease in bilirubin (LEITE, 2004).

According to Barbosa (1988):

> There is no precise limit for each session, however, as the child will most often be taken out of the system to be breastfed, the

rest period between feeds can be used as exposure time (BARBOSA, 1988, p. 127).

The maximum bilirubin level is usually reached on the 3rd or 4th day of life in term neonates. In preterm babies, the maximum level is not reached until the end of the first week. Phototherapy should be definitively withdrawn when, after its suspension, the newborn continues to show a drop in the serum bilirubin level (LEITE, 2004).

Types of phototherapy:

CONVENTIONAL PHOTOTHERAPY

According to Carvalho (2001), common or conventional phototherapy consists of six to seven lamps. The body surface area illuminated is large, since the whole newborn is irradiated by the light.

For Correa and Tomasi (2008),

> In conventional phototherapy, white light has been the most widely used over the years and is the only type of light whose safety has been tested on a large population of newborns monitored during the first six years of life (CORREA and TOMASI, 2008, p. 5).

BILISPOT PHOTOTHERAPY

According to Carvalho (2001) there is also Bilispot Phototherapy, as the name suggests, the light is emitted in the form of a spot or focus.

Campos (2008) states that,

The irradiance of Bilisport Phototherapy is much higher than that emitted by conventional phototherapies. It uses halogen-tungsten lamps that produce a high emission, in the blue range of 25 to 30 pW/cm^2 /nm, and with filters for ultraviolet and infrared radiation, but unlike conventional phototherapy, it is uneven in its distribution with a very large central concentration peak. When placed at a distance of 40-50cm from the newborn, it provides a luminous halo 20cm in diameter with a high irradiance in the centre, and as it moves to the periphery, it drops sharply. For small newborns, this type of light is extremely effective as it illuminates their body surface with considerable irradiance (CAMPOS apud CORREA and TOMASI, 2008, p. 6).

BILIBID PHOTOTHERAPY

Bilibid phototherapy is most commonly used for large newborns, where fluorescent lamps are used under an acrylic cradle. According to Murahovschi (2008), this type of phototherapy aims to:

To avoid losing rays from below, reflective film can be placed on the side walls and top dome of the newborn. In this way, it will receive light from below and indirectly from above, and from the sides, which in addition to increasing the irradiance of conventional phototherapy, will increase light exposure (MURAHOVSCHI apud CORREA and TOMASI, 2008, p. 6-7).

OCTOPHOTO PHOTOTHERAPY

The Octofoto has a steel plate, the edges of which are finished in textured epoxy® paint. The reflector system is made of moulded plastic material and is attached to a "T" shaped pedestal with 2" swivel castors, which makes it easier to move and with a variable height that can be adjusted by locking it using a clamp system (ROSSI FILHO, 2007).

NURSING CARE FOR NEWBORNS
BEING TREATED WITH PHOTOTHERAPY

Newborn care is divided into immediate and general care. Immediate care is care that the team must take in the delivery room to maintain the life of the newborn and avoid future sequelae, while general care is care during the neonatal period, when the child is adapting to life outside the womb (ORLANDI and SABRÁ, 2005).

Nursing has a wide-ranging role, from fully identifying the components, handling, choosing, adapting, adjusting and measuring the irradiance of the devices with or without the baby, to specifically caring for the newborn undergoing phototherapy in order to obtain the best results, in the shortest time and with the fewest acceptable side effects in this practice (GAÍVA, GOMES, 2003).

It is up to the nursing team to be familiar with these procedures in order not only to fulfil the prescription, but also to care for the jaundiced newborn with knowledge, safety, efficiency and special care to achieve the results (CAMPOS, MOREIRA, 2006).

Subjecting NBs to phototherapy interrupts the mother-child emotional bond, as it is a treatment that requires specific care and guidance for the carer and especially for mothers, who are extremely important co-participants in NB care (RODRIGUES; SILVEIRA; CAMPOS, 2007).

According to Gomes, Teixeira and Barichello (2010), NBs undergoing phototherapy require special care from a multi-professional team and nurses, as the link in this team, are responsible for 24-hour care and must be trained to diagnose complications and intervene quickly and efficiently.

Therefore, all health professionals who handle phototherapy must be familiarised with the rules, existing routines and the functioning of the equipment, aware of the need to adhere to them and qualified to apply them, as well as regularly evaluating the efficiency and effectiveness of this therapeutic modality (VIEIRA et al., 2004).

The necessary care for NBs during phototherapy treatment is to keep them unclothed and wearing eye protection; change their position; carry out a water balance; observe eliminations; check irradiance; carry out temperature control and observe changes to the skin due to the risk of burns (ABREU; NASCIMENTO, 2008).

The body surface area should be as large as possible, and the NB should remain without clothes and preferably without a nappy (BUENO, SACAI, TOMA, 2003; CORREA, TOMASI, 2007). However, as many newborns have diarrhoeal bowel movements due to the treatment itself, it is not always possible to keep them without a nappy.

Eye protection is mandatory to prevent exposure to light. It should be done with an opaque blindfold, of an appropriate size and positioned to completely cover the eyes, but without occluding the nostrils. The eyelids should be closed before putting on the mask to prevent corneal abrasions and eye hygiene should be carried out with saline solution (BUENO, SACAI, TOMA, 2003; CORREA, TOMASI, 2007). During breastfeeding, it is recommended that the blindfold be removed to allow the opportunity for visual and sensory stimuli and thus establish the mother-child bond.

In addition to this, other basic care should be given to the newborn during phototherapy, including: measuring daily weight and carrying out a rigorous water balance, due to the increased insensible losses; increasing water intake, preferably via the enteric route, using breast milk or appropriate milk formulas; checking vital signs every 2 hours, paying greater attention to temperature, due to the tendency to hyperthermia and the risk of overheating; not using ointments, oils and creams, due to the risk of

burns on the neonate's skin (BUENO, SACAI, TOMA, 2003; COLVERO, COLVERO, FIORI, 2005; CORREA, TOMASI, 2007).

However, for this treatment to be administered, the NB needs to be hospitalised, which can directly affect the bond between mother and child. While for many health professionals phototherapy is a simple and routine treatment, for mothers it can seem like a strange, unknown and even frightening treatment. Some professionals don't realise that this treatment arouses such feelings, as it is a non-invasive treatment (CAMPOS, CARDOSO, 2004).

According to Rosa and Furlanetto (2012), decubitus changes prevent complications by maintaining skin integrity and avoiding overheating.

Colvero, Colvero and Fiori (2005) state that the NB should ideally be changed decubitus every two hours to increase the area of exposure. According to Kenner (2001), this change also relieves pressure on the knees, hips and other joints and should be carried out whenever necessary, often before 2 hours.

There is disagreement between some authors about the time interval for taking the temperature. While Cloherty and Stark (1993), Campos and Cardoso (2004) and Tamez and Silva (2009) indicate that temperature should preferably be taken in the axillary region every 2 hours, Gomes, Teixeira and Barichello (2010) state that it should be checked every 2-4 hours and Simões (2002) describes that temperature control should be carried out every 4 hours or at shorter intervals if necessary.

Given the importance of this check for the neonate's health, it should be carried out every 2 hours to identify possible thermal alterations, which can be intervened upon more quickly, thus enabling adequate care for the NB. It is advised that the check be carried out with the device switched off and the NB out of the device to avoid errors (OLIVEIRA et al., 2011).

With regard to hydration conditions, a water balance should be taken and recorded, the skin and mucous membranes should be weighed, assessed and recorded,

as well as the appearance and quantity of physiological eliminations and the characteristics of the fontanels (GOMES; TEIXEIRA; BARICHELLO, 2010). This assessment is important because NBs undergoing
Phototherapy has a risk of developing dehydration as a result of insensible losses and diarrhoea (TAMEZ; SILVA, 2009).

To keep a child nourished and hydrated, Simões (2002) says that breastfeeding should be encouraged. Professionals need to help mothers with breastfeeding techniques, encourage more frequent feeds of at least eight times a day and make sure that the NB takes the amount of artificial food provided (MARTÍNEZ et al., 2011).

If the NB is excessively jaundiced and the cause of the jaundice is breastfeeding, Cloherty and Stark (1993) report that breastfeeding should be temporarily suspended until bilirubin levels normalise. During this period, the NB should be fed appropriate formula.

With regard to observing and recording adverse events and preventing complications, it is important for nursing professionals to carry out this care, because NBs exposed to phototherapy may present some alterations that must be prevented and detected early by the nursing team, in order to provide effective results and guarantee treatment efficacy.

Despite its beneficial effects in the treatment of neonatal hyperbilirubinaemia, phototherapy is not without its risks. [a]There are some complications from its use, although they are minor compared to those that the neonate would experience without its use, such as: insensible water loss, an increase in the number of bowel movements, changes in red blood cells, lethargy, erythema, slower growth in infancy, tanning, burns and the possibility of retinal damage (CAMPOS; CARDOSO, 2004).

Gomes, Teixeira and Barichello (2010) add other reactions of NB exposed to light: diarrhoea; susceptibility to hyperthermia and hypothermia due to direct exposure to the heat source or lack of heating when in a common cot or bib; skin rashes and erythema; darkening of the skin called tanned baby syndrome; burns; mild haemolysis; thrombocytopenia and retinal damage.

Other complications were mentioned in the study by Colovero, Colvero and Fiori (2005): genotoxicity; thermal instability; skin rash; hypocalcaemia; abdominal distension; increased respiratory and heart rate; irritability and aerophagia due to occlusion of the eyes.

In their study, Campos and Cardoso (2004) also identified adverse effects on NB mothers, who were upset when they saw their child undergoing phototherapy, particularly because of the occlusion of the eyes. The treatment can also interfere with the bonding process of the mother-child dyad, breaking the bond and generating anxiety.

CONCLUSION

This study on newborns undergoing phototherapy concluded that despite the inclusion criteria, the number of studies found in the survey was low, describing the main nursing care for newborns undergoing phototherapy: protecting the eyes with an appropriate blindfold; strict water balance; checking vital signs every two hours; changing position at least every four hours; not using oils or moisturising creams; checking irradiance and promoting the mother-child bond. We can see that it is essential for nursing professionals to develop new actions in order to improve the quality of care, including guidance and communication between the health team and mothers of newborns undergoing phototherapy treatment, so that they are aware of the disease, the treatment, its benefits and risks and can feel at ease while carrying out the appropriate care for their children undergoing phototherapy treatment.

The most likely reason for this may be the difficulty in publicising nurses' actions. Some studies indicate that the lack of ability to write and publicise their professional experiences, the low consumption of scientific research results, the lack of support and guidance in this area, as well as the lack of encouragement from employers are some of the difficulties reported by nursing assistants in developing and publishing scientific work.

REFERENCES

Campos ACS, Cardoso MVLM, Pagliuca LMF, Rossi LA. Communication: a basic nursing tool for caring for the mother of a neonate under phototherapy. Journal of the Northeast Nursing Network. Fortaleza. 2008.

Campos ACS, Cardoso MVLML. Application of Paterson and Zderad's theory with mothers of newborns under phototherapy. Texto Contexto Enferm ; 13(3):435-43 Fortaleza - CE.2004.

Campos ACS, Cardoso MVLML. Nursing and humanistic care: an intervention proposal for the mother of a neonate under phototherapy. Fortaleza-CE. Ciencia y Enfermeria. 2006.

Campos ACS, Cardoso MVLML. The newborn under phototherapy: The mother's perception. Rev latino-am Enfermagem. 2004.

Campos ACS, Cardoso MVLML. Educational technology for the practice of nursing care with mothers of neonates under phototherapy. Texto Contexto Enfermagem. Florianópolis. 2008.

Carvalho M. Lopes JMA. Indications for phototherapy in term newborns with non-hemolytic jaundice: a critical analysis. Journal of Paediatrics. Rio de Janeiro. 1995.

Cestari TF, Pressato S, Corrêa GP. Phototherapy - clinical applications. An Brasileiros de Dermatologia. Porto Alegre - RS, 82(1):5-6. 2007.

De Carvalho M. Treatment of neonatal jaundice. Journal of Paediatrics. Rio de Janeiro.2001.

Duarte I, Buense R, Kobata C. Phototherapy. Anais Brasileiros de Demartologia. 2006.

Facchini FP, Mezzacappa MA, Rosa IR, et al. Follow-up of jaundice in term and late preterm neonates. J Paediatria. Rio de Janeiro .83(4):313-318.2007

Gomes NS, Teixeira JBA, Barichello E. Care of the newborn in phototherapy: the knowledge of the nursing team. Revista Eletronica de Enfermagem. 2010.

Martins BMR, Carvalho M, Moreira MEL, Lopes JMA. Evaluation of the clinical efficacy of a new phototherapy modality using light-emitting diodes. Journal of Paediatrics. Rio de Janeiro. 2007.

Pimpão FD, Kerber NC, Francioni FF, Rangel RF, Filho WDL. Nursing care in rooming-in: An integrative review. Cogitare Enferm. 2010.

Punaro E, Mezzacappa MA, Facchini FP. Systematised monitoring of hyperbilirubinaemia in newborns between 35 and 37 weeks of gestational age. J Pediatria. Rio Janeiro. 2011;87(4):301-6.

Silva I, Luco M, Tapia JL, et al. Single versus double phototherapy in the treatment of term newborns with nonhaemolytic hyperbilirubinaemia. J. Paediatria. Rio de Janeiro. 85(5):455-458.2009.

Vasconcelos CKB, Bianchi RF. Luminescent polymers as non-ionising radiation sensors: Application in neonatal phototherapy. Polymers: science and technology. Ouro Preto - MG, v.17,n.4,p. 325-328. 2007.

Vieira AA, Lima CLMA, Carvalho M, Moreira MEL. The use of phototherapy in newborns: evaluation of clinical practice. Brazilian Journal of Maternal and Child

Health. Recife, 4(4).2004.

41

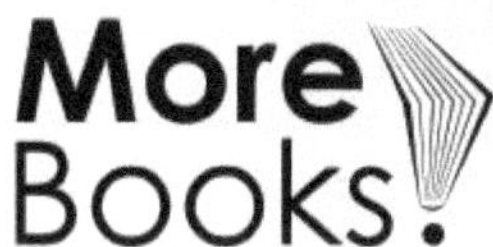

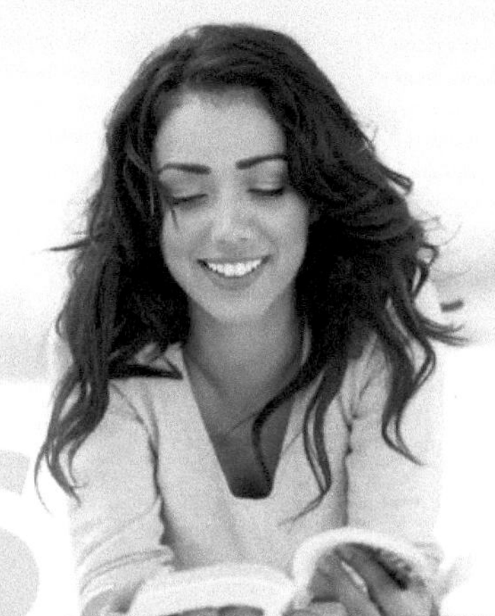

I want morebooks!

Buy your books fast and straightforward online - at one of world's fastest growing online book stores! Environmentally sound due to Print-on-Demand technologies.

Buy your books online at
www.morebooks.shop

Kaufen Sie Ihre Bücher schnell und unkompliziert online – auf einer der am schnellsten wachsenden Buchhandelsplattformen weltweit! Dank Print-On-Demand umwelt- und ressourcenschonend produziert.

Bücher schneller online kaufen
www.morebooks.shop

info@omniscriptum.com
www.omniscriptum.com

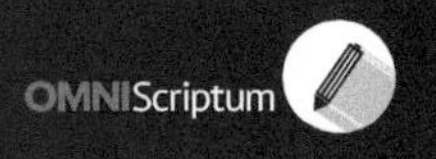